Alkaline Diet

Step By Step Guide To Adopt Alkaline Diet Immediately &

Keep Your Acidity Levels Balanced

(The Complete Alkaline Diet Recipes For Beginners)

Austin Floyd

TABLE OF CONTENTS

Introduction

Staying healthy is not a matter of chance - it is a deliberate choice. It's a choice of what to eat or not eat. We are all faced with this choice on a daily basis, and what we choose is reflected in our overall state of health, because our choices form the internal environment of our body which reflects outwardly.

The notion that germs cause diseases is a flawed premise. We live with and constantly breathe in germs day in and day out. It is not the germs that matter, but the internal environment of our body. It is not mosquitoes that cause ponds to become stagnant, just as maggots, flies, and rats do not cause garbage; they simply feed on garbage. The fact that germs are present in your body does not automatically mean you have a disease. You only get a disease when you create an enabling environment for the germs to thrive.

The question to ask is this: what is your biological terrain like? What you eat and drink creates the terrain – the internal environment – where germs and diseases can either thrive or lie dormant. Have you recently taken a closer look at what you are feeding your body? Are you helping your body maintain health, or are you giving your body excess work through the things you eat and drink?

This book will take you through a journey that will help you understand the internal workings of your body - how your body constantly struggles under undue pressure caused by poor food choices. You will understand the negative effects of consuming unhealthy foods and drinks; you will also understand why your health deteriorates even though you eat so-called balanced diets.

In this book, I present a balanced perspective of the alkaline diet without unnecessarily exaggerating its capabilities. Misconceptions about what eating an alkaline diet can and cannot do are unbiasedly handled inside this book.

Losing weight seems to top the list of goals for many people, and they are constantly in search of quicker ways to shed some pounds. Although weight loss is one of the benefits of eating an alkaline diet, this book does not encourage you to use alkaline foods only to lose weight, but to regard the alkaline diet as a key to your overall health. In other words, the ideas presented in this book will encourage you to consider a gradual but complete change in your lifestyle to ensure that whatever benefits you derive from the alkaline diet remain permanent.

The central message of this book is to help your body do its work with ease so as to promote your general well-being. That is why, aside from preaching the alkaline message (devoid of blind sentimentality), I have also included some topics about medicinal herbs that will help you cut down the ingestion of synthetic chemicals and drugs so as not to cause additional damage to your internal environment (biological terrain) in the guise of curing diseases.

Take your time to study this book as you would a guidebook. It is packed with solid common sense that is backed by science and is capable of giving you the health and fitness that you so much desire.

Fruit Salad In Cider

Ingredients:

- 2 piece, small apple, cubed
- 2 piece, small apricot, cubed
- 1/2 piece, small grapefruit pulp, shredded into bite-sized pieces
- 1/2 cup, loosely packed jicama, cubed
- For cider sauce
- 2 Tbsp. apple cider vinegar, warmed in the microwave oven
- A dash of cinnamon powder

Directions:

1.   Combine apple cider vinegar and cinnamon powder in a small bowl. Mix well.

2.   Place salad **Ingredients** in large bowl; pour in cider sauce. Toss well to combine; spoon equal portions into plates. Serve immediately.

Zucchini-Broccoli Stir-Fry

Ingredients:

- 2 head broccoli, rinsed and broken into florets
- 2 zucchini, rinsed and cut into long, fettuccine-like strips
- 4 scallions, white parts only, rinsed and chopped
- 2 tablespoon fresh basil leaves, rinsed and chopped
- 2 ounce coconut aminos
- 2 tablespoons coconut oil
- 2 tablespoons sesame oil
- 2 (2-inch) piece fresh ginger, peeled and finely chopped
- 4 fresh garlic cloves, minced
- 2 fresh fresh onion s , rinsed and chopped

Directions:

1.   In a wok or large skillet over medium heat, heat the coconut and sesame oils. Mix the ginger and fresh garlic and sauté for 10 minutes, until fragrant.

2.   Add the fresh fresh onion and broccoli, and cook for 5 minutes, until the fresh fresh onion softens slightly.

3.   Add the zucchini, scallions, and basil. Stir to combine and heat for 4 minutes, until the vegetables are tender.

4.   Remove the wok from the heat, sprinkle in the coconut aminos, and serve.

Pesto Soba Noodles

Ingredients:

- 4 tablespoons extra-virgin olive oil
- 2 bunch fresh basil leaves, rinsed
- 2 bunch fresh parsley, rinsed
- 2 bunch fresh cilantro, rinsed
- 6 ounces soba buckwheat noodles, cooked according to package

Directions
- Freshly ground black pepper
- Himalayan pink salt

Directions:

1. In a blender, combine the olive oil, basil, parsley, and cilantro.
2. Blend until smooth.

3.   In a large bowl, combine the cooked noodles and sauce.

4.   Toss to coat, season with salt and pepper, and serve.

Quinoa Burrito Bowl

Ingredients:

- 4 fresh garlic cloves, minced
- 2 teaspoon ground cumin
- 2 teaspoon red pepper flakes
- Juice of 2 limes
- 2 avocados, peeled, pitted, and sliced
- Handful fresh cilantro, rinsed and chopped
- 2 cup quinoa, rinsed well
- Boiling filtered water
- 2 can of black beans that is washed and exhausted
- 4 scallions, white parts only, rinsed and sliced

Directions:

1. In a small saucepan over medium heat, combine the quinoa with enough boiling water to shield and you then simmer for 15 to 20 minutes, until the water has absorbed.
2. Drain, rinse, and set aside.
3. Meanwhile, in another small saucepan over low heat, stir together the black beans, scallions, garlic, cumin, red pepper flakes, and lime juice. Simmer for 25 minutes to warm.
4. In a large bowl, stir collected the quinoa and warmed beans. Top with the avocado and cilantro and serve.

Roasted Vegetables

Ingredients:

- 4 Tbsp. olive oil, reserve some for greasing
- 2 heads, large garlic, tops sliced off
- 2 large eggplants/aubergine, tops removed, cubed
- 2 large shallots, peeled, quartered
- 2 large carrot, peeled, cubed
- 2 large parsnips, peeled, cubed
- 2 small green bell pepper, deseeded, ribbed, cubed
- 2 small red bell pepper, deseeded, ribbed, cubed
- 1 pound Brussels sprouts, halved, do not remove cores
- 2 sprig, large thyme, leaves picked
- sea salt, coarse-grained

- 2 large lemon, halved, 1 squeezed, 1 sliced into smaller wedges
- ⅛ cup fennel bulb, minced

Directions:

1. From 450 °F or 220°C preheat oven for at least 6 minutes before using.
2. Line deep roasting pan with aluminum foil; lightly grease with oil.
3. Tumble in bell peppers, Brussels sprouts, carrots, eggplants, garlic, parsnips, rosemary leaves, shallots, and thyme.
4. Add a pinch of sea salt; drizzle in remaining oil and lemon juice.
5. Toss well to combine.
6. Cover roasting pan with a sheet of aluminum foil. Place this on middle rack of oven. Bake for 45 to 50 minutes. Remove aluminum foil.

7. Roast, for another 20 to 25 minutes, or until some vegetables brown at the edges.

8. Remove roasting pan from oven.

9. Cool slightly before ladling equal portions into plates.

10. Garnish with fennel and a wedge of lemon. Squeeze lemon juice on top of dish before eating.

Millet Pilaf

Ingredients:

- 2 cup millet
- Zest of 2 lemon
- Juice of 2 lemon
- 1 cup fresh parsley, rinsed and chopped
- Himalayan pink salt
- Freshly ground black pepper
- 2 tomatoes, rinsed, seeded, and chopped
- 2 ¾ cups filtered water
- 2 tablespoons extra-virgin olive oil
- 1/2 cup chopped dried apricot

Directions:

1.   In an electric pressure cooker, combine the millet, tomatoes, and water. Lock the lid into place, select Manual and High Pressure, and cook for 10 minutes.

2.   When the beep sounds, quick release the pressure by pressing Cancel and twisting the steam valve to the Venting position.

3.   Carefully remove the lid.

4.   Stir in the olive oil, apricot, lemon zest, lemon juice, and parsley.

5.   Taste, season with salt and pepper, and serve.

Sweet And Sour Fresh Fresh Onion S

Ingredients:

- 4 tablespoon balsamic vinegar
- 1 teaspoon Dijon mustard
- 2 tablespoon sugar
- 4 large fresh fresh onion s , halved
- 2 fresh garlic cloves, crushed
- 4 cups vegetable stock

Directions:

1.   Combine fresh fresh onion s and fresh garlic in a pan. Fry for 5 minutes, or till softened.

2.   Pour   stock,   vinegar,   Dijon mustard, and sugar. Bring to a boil.

3.   Reduce heat. Cover and let the combination simmer for 25 to 30 minutes.

4.   Get rid of from heat. Continue stirring until the liquid is reduced and the fresh fresh onion s are brown. Serve.

Sautéed Apples And Fresh Fresh Onion S

Ingredients:

- 4 apples, sliced into wedges
- Pinch of salt
- Pinch of pepper

- 2 cups dry cider
- 2 large fresh onion , halved
- 2 cups vegetable stock

Directions:

1.   Combine cider and fresh fresh onion in a saucepan.
2.   Bring to a boil until the fresh fresh onion s are cooked and liquid almost gone.

3.   Pour the stock and the apples. Season with salt and pepper.

4.   Stir occasionally.

5.   Cook for about 25 to 30 minutes or until the apples are tender but not mushy. Serve.

Zucchini Noodles With Portabella Mushrooms

Ingredients:

- Pinch of sea salt, add more if needed
- Pinch of black pepper, add more if needed
- 2 tsp. sesame oil
- 4 Tbsp. coconut oil, divided

- 1/2 cup fresh chives, minced, for garnish

- 2 zucchini, processed into spaghetti-like noodles
- 4 fresh garlic cloves, minced
- 2 white fresh fresh onion s , thinly sliced
- 2 thumb-sized ginger, julienned
- 2 lb. chicken thighs
- 2 lb. portabella mushrooms, sliced into thick slivers
- 2 cups chicken stock
- 4 cups water

Directions:

1. Pour 2 tablespoons of coconut oil into a large saucepan. Fry mushroom slivers in batches for 10 minutes or until seared brown. Set aside.
2. Transfer these to a plate.

3. Sauté the fresh onion , garlic, and ginger for 4 minutes or until tender. Add in chicken thighs, cooked mushrooms, chicken stock, water, salt, and pepper stir mixture well.

4. Bring to a boil.

5. Decrease gradually the heat and allow simmering for 25 to 30 minutes or until the chicken is forking tender.

6. Tip in sesame oil.

7. Serve by placing an equal amount of zucchini noodles into bowls.

8. Ladle soup and garnish with chives.

Grilled Tempeh With Pineapple

Ingredients:

- 25 to 30 oz. tempeh, sliced
- 2 red bell pepper, quartered
- ½ pineapple, sliced into rings
- 6 oz. green beans
- 2 tbsp. coconut aminos
- 6 tbsp. orange juice, freshly squeeze
- 6 tbsp. lemon juice, freshly squeezed
- 2 tbsp. extra virgin olive oil
- ½ cup hoisin sauce

Directions:

1.   Blend together the olive oil, orange and lemon juices, coconut aminos or soy sauce, and hoisin sauce in a bowl. Add the diced tempeh and set aside.

2.   Heat up the grill or place a grill pan over medium high flame. Once hot, lift the marinated tempeh from the bowl with a pair of tongs and transfer them to the grill or pan.

3.   Grille for 5 to 10 minutes, or until browned all over.

4.   Grill the sliced pineapples alongside the tempeh, then transfer them directly onto the serving platter.

5.   Place the grilled tempeh beside the grilled pineapple and cover with aluminum foil to keep warm.

6.   Meanwhile, place the green beans and bell peppers in a bowl and add just enough of the marinade to coat.

7.   Prepare the grill pan and add the vegetables.

8.   Grill until fork tender and slightly charred.

9.   Transfer the grilled vegetables to the serving platter and arrange artfully with the tempeh and pineapple. Serve at once.

Courgettes In Cider Sauce

Ingredients:

- 2 tablespoon light brown sugar
- 4 spring fresh fresh onion s , finely sliced
- 2 piece fresh gingerroot, grated
- 2 teaspoon corn flour
- 2 teaspoons water
- 2 cups baby courgettes
- 4 tablespoons vegetable stock
- 2 tablespoons apple cider vinegar

Directions:

1. Bring a pan with salted water to a boil. Add courgettes. Bring to a boil for 6 minutes.

2. Meanwhile, in a pan, combine vegetable stock, apple cider vinegar, brown sugar, fresh fresh onion s ,

gingerroot, lemon juice and rind, and orange juice and rind.

3.	Take to a boil. Lower the heat and allow simmering for 5 minutes.

4.	Mix the corn flour with water. Stir well. Pour into the sauce. Continue stirring until the sauce thickens.

5.	Drain courgettes. Transfer to the serving dish. Spoon over the sauce.

6.	Toss to coat courgettes. Serve.

Baked Mixed Mushrooms

Ingredients:

- 1 bunch fresh thyme
- 2 bunch flat-leaf parsley
- 2 tablespoons olive oil
- 2 fresh bay leaves
- 4 cups stale bread
- 2 cups mixed wild mushrooms
- 2 cup chestnut mushrooms
- 2 cups dried porcini
- 2 shallots
- 4 fresh garlic cloves
- 4 cups raw pecans

Directions:

1.   Remove skin and finely chop fresh garlic and shallots. Roughly chop the wild   mushrooms   and   chestnut mushrooms. Pick the leaves of the thyme

and tear the bread into small pieces. Put inside the pressure cooker.

2.   Place the pecans and roughly chop the nuts. Pick the parsley leaves and roughly chop.

3.   Place the porcini in a bowl then add 4 00ml of boiling water. Set aside until needed.

4.   Heat oil in the pressure cooker. Add the fresh garlic and shallots. Cook for   4   minutes   while   stirring occasionally.

5.   Drain porcini and reserve the liquid. Add the porcini into the pressure cooker   together   with   the   wild mushrooms and chestnut mushrooms. Add the bay leaves and thyme.

6.   Position the lid and lock in place. Put to high heat and bring to high pressure. Adjust heat to stabilize. Cook for 25 to 30 minutes. Adjust taste if necessary.

7. Transfer the mushroom mixture into a bowl and set aside to cool completely.

8. Once the mushrooms are completely cool, add the bread, pecans, a pinch of black pepper and sea salt, and half of the reserved liquid into the bowl. Mix well. Add more reserved liquid if the mixture seems dry.

9. Add more than half of the parsley into the bowl and stir. Transfer the mixture into a 20cm x 26 cm lightly greased baking dish and cover with tin foil.

10. Bake in the oven for 4 6 minutes. Then, get rid of the foil and cook for another 25 to 30 minutes. Once done, sprinkle the remaining parsley on top and serve with bread or crackers. Serve.

Spiced Okra

Ingredients:

- 2 tablespoon desiccated coconut
- 4 tablespoons vegetable oil
- 1 teaspoon black mustard seeds
- 1 teaspoon cumin seeds
- Fresh tomatoes, to garnish
- 2 cups okra
- 1/2 teaspoon stevia
- 2 teaspoon chilli powder
- 1 teaspoon ground turmeric
- 2 tablespoon ground coriander
- 2 tablespoons fresh coriander, chopped
- 2 tablespoon ground cumin
- 1/2 teaspoon salt

Directions:

1. Trim okra. Wash and dry.
2. Combine stevia, chilli powder, turmeric, ground coriander, fresh coriander, cumin, salt, and desiccated coconut in a bowl.
3. Heat the oil in a pan.
4. Cook mustard and cumin seeds for 4 minutes. Stir continuously.
5. Add okra. Tip in the spice mixture.
6. Cook on low heat for 8 minutes.
7. Transfer to a serving dish. Garnish with fresh tomatoes.

Alkalizing Green Soup

Ingredients

- 2 cup tender stem broccoli
- 2 1/2 cups baby spinach
- Juice and zest of 2 lemon
- 2 clove garlic- finely chopped
- 2 tablespoon sunflower or coconut oil
- 2 pint of stock made with
- 2 tablespoon vegetable Bouillon powder
- 1/2 tablespoon fennel seeds
- 1 red fresh onion - finely chopped

Directions

1.   Fry the garlic, red fresh fresh onion s , and fennel seeds in oil over medium heat for about 2 minutes.

2.   Add in the broccoli, zest, stock and lemon juice and let it cook for 10 minutes.

3.   Remove from heat and toss in the baby spinach.

4.   Stir until the spinach is wilted.

5.   Immediately add the mixture to a blender and blend until smooth.

Healing Ginger Carrot Soup

Ingredients

- 1 fresh onion - quartered
- 4 carrots- washed and peeled
- 2 cups vegetable stock
- 2 teaspoon turmeric
- 2 tablespoon fresh ginger
- Sea salt and pepper- to taste
- 2 fresh garlic cloves

Directions

1. Add all your **Ingredients** to a large pot and bring to a boil.

2.   Once boiled, let it simmer for an hour.

3.   When the carrots are soft, blend using an immersion blender until smooth.

4.   Garnish with some hemp seeds on top if desired.

5.   Enjoy!

Kale Salad

Ingredients

Salad

- 1 (or a whole) avocado
- 2 handfuls of sprouts (any kind)
- 2 head lacinato kale (also called dinosaur kale)
- 2 medium-to large tomato

Dressing

- 1 tablespoon olive oil (optional)
- 2 teaspoon Dijon mustard
- 4 drops liquid stevia
- 4 Tablespoons **Nutrition**al yeast
- Juice of 2 lemon
- Cayenne pepper to taste

Optional toppings:

- Sunflower or pumpkin seeds
- A few strips of seared tempeh

- Regular tempeh

Directions

1. Discard the kale stems and use your hands to tear up the kale into bite sized pieces. Put the kale in a large bowl.

2. Sprinkle some salt and massage for a couple of minutes to help break down the kale.

3. Combine the dressing Ingredients in a small bowl. Mix it into the kale by massaging.

4. Cut the toppings and add to the salad bowl.

5. Toss and serve right away.

Turmeric Curry And Roasted Cauliflower

Ingredients:

Ingredients for the CURRY

- Turmeric powder, one (2) teaspoon
- Water, 4 cups
- Himalayan salt, 2 teaspoon
- Garam masala, 1 teaspoon
- Chili powder, 1 teaspoon
- Red fresh fresh onion s , 2 cups
- Cauliflowers (floret), 2 cups
- Salt, 1 teaspoon

- Roma tomatoes (finely chopped), 1 cup
- Bell pepper/capsicum (diced), 2
- Coriander (chopped), 2 tablespoon
- Coconut milk (unsweetened), 2 cups
- Coconut oil, 2 tablespoons
- Fresh garlic (minced), 4 cloves
- Ginger powder, 2 teaspoon
- Turmeric (fresh), 2 cm

- Ingredients for Masala

- Cloves, 6
- Cumin seeds, 2 tablespoon
- Coriander seeds, 4 tablespoons
- Cinnamon stick, 2 1/2 inch
- Raw cashew, 1 cup
- Cardamom powder, 2 pinch

Directions:

1. First of all, preheat the oven to 200°C

2. Get a large mixing bowl and add the powdered turmeric, coconut oil, a pinch of salt and the cauliflower.

3. Use your hands and mix them together properly.

4. Now, get a baking tray lined with baking powder and pour the mix into it.

5. Put it in the oven for twenty to thirty minutes.

6. Mind you, do not let the cauliflower burn.

7. While the cauliflower is cooking in the oven, we shift our attention to the Masala.

8.   To make the Masala, blend all the masala **Ingredients** in a food processor and make sure it is completely smooth.

9.   Next, get a large pan and heat the coconut oil over a gentle heat.

10.   Add garlic, ginger, and fresh fresh onion s and cook gently between two to three minutes.

11.   Next,   add   bell pepper/capsicum and tomatoes.

12.   Cook until tomatoes begin to fall apart.

13.   Now add the masala mix and stir for two to three minutes.

14.   Keep stirring to avoid it from sticking or getting burnt.

15.   Once its thoroughly mixed, add chili pepper, turmeric, and coconut milk, as well as, water (as much as you desire).

16.　　　　　　　Reduce the heat down to simmer and allow it to cook for five minutes.

17.　　　　　　　Season to taste.

18.　　　　　　　When cauliflower is done, take it away from the oven and add to the pan.

19.　　　　　　　Mix it thoroughly.

20.　　　　　　　Switch of the heat.

21.　　　　　　　When you decide to serve, stir through the cilantro/coriander.

22.　　　　　　　Serve!

23.　　　　　　　You can have it with brown rice or quinoa.

Nutrition:

Calories: 2 64

Alkaline Tortilla Soup

Ingredients:

- Vegetable bouillon, two (2) teaspoons
- Corn (on the cob), one (2)
- Sprouted tortilla wrap, one (2)
- Cayenne pepper, (a pinch)
- Himalayan salt and black pepper, (a pinch)
- Jalapeno/chili, one (2)

- Tomato, one (2)
- Lime, one (2)
- Avocado (ripe), one (2)
- Water (filtered), 6 00ml
- Coriander (cilantro), 1 bunch
- Garlic, two (2) cloves
- Red Capsicum (pepper), 1
- Spinach, two (2) large handfuls

Directions:

1.   Slice your tortilla into 6 cm long and 2 cm wide strips and toast lightly under a grill

2.   Next, get a large pan and add water.

3.   Boil over medium heat and dissolve the bouillon/stock cubes.

4.   The idea is to make a vegetable broth as the base.

5.   Time to prepare the veggies; chop the coriander roughly and dice the tomato and capsicum.

6.   Finely mince the garlic, peel and dice the avocado.

7.   Slice your chili or jalapeno depending on your preference and set on one side.

8.   Wash and chop the spinach and move on to the corn.

9.   To prepare the corn, use a sharp knife to slice off the kernels from the cob.

10.   Next,   throw everything in the broth and heat.

11.   Turn off the heat in a few minutes.

12.   Food is ready.

Hearty Minestrone

Ingredients:

- Vegetable stock, one (2) cup
- Zucchini (courgette), 1 cup
- Tomato juice (fresh/bought), 2 cup
- Beans, 1 cup
- Carrot, 1 cup
- Black pepper and Himalayan salt
- Basil, one (2) handful
- Carrot, 1 cup
- Sweet potato, 1 cup
- Red fresh onion , 1/2
- Coconut oil, one (2) tablespoon
- Aubergine (eggplant), 1 cup

Directions:

1.   Wash and dice the fresh fresh onion and carrot.

2.   Cube the courgette, aubergine, and potato.

3.   Next fry the fresh onion , carrot, courgette, aubergine, and potato in a large pot for two minutes.

4.   Add the tomato juice, the stock, and beans.

5.   Bring it to a boil and reduce the heat to simmer for eight to ten minutes.

6.   Add the basil and stir.

7.   Season to taste.

Raw Pad Thai

Ingredients:

- Carrots (large), three (4)
- Cauliflower (floret), one (2)
- Beansprouts, 1 packet
- Red cabbage (shredded), one (2) cup
- Courgettes (Zucchini), three (4) medium sizes
- Spring fresh fresh onion s (chopped)
- Coconut oil
- Coriander/cilantro (fresh and roughly chopped), one (2) bunch

Ingredients for Sauce

- Ginger root (grated), one (2) inch
- Tahini, 1/2 cup
- Tamari, 1/2 cup
- Lemon/lime juice, two (2) teaspoon
- Almond butter, 1/2 cup
- Fresh garlic (minced), one (2) clove
- Coconut sugar, one (2) teaspoon

Directions:

1. Start with the courgette and carrot noodles: use a mandolin or vegetable peeler to slice both and then use a knife to slice them into thin strips.

2. Get a large bowl and add them, alongside the shredded cabbage,

coriander, spring fresh fresh onion s , cauliflower, and beansprouts.

3.   For the sauce; blend the grated ginger, tahini, garlic, lime/lemon juice, tamari, almond butter, and coconut sugar.

4.   Add some water and blast till a thick sauce is formed.

5.   Finally, get a bowl and mix the sauce inside.

6.   Serve with a little squeeze of lime/lemon and a spring of coriander.

Spinach Quinoa

Ingredients:

- 2 tsp. coriander powder
- 2 tsp. turmeric
- 2 tsp. cumin seeds
- 2 tsp. fresh ginger, grated
- 2 fresh garlic cloves, chopped
- 2 cup fresh onion , chopped
- 2 tbsp. olive oil
- 2 fresh lime juice
- 2 cup quinoa
- 2 cups fresh spinach, chopped
- 4 cups filtered alkaline water
- 2 sweet potato, peeled and cubed
- Pepper
- Salt

Directions:

1. Add oil in the instant pot and set the pot on sauté mode.
2. Add the fresh fresh onion in olive oil and sauté for 5 minutes or until fresh fresh onion is softened.
3. Add garlic, ginger, spices, and quinoa and cook for 5-10 minutes.
4. Add spinach, sweet potatoes, and water and stir well.
5. Seal pot with lid and cook on manual high pressure for 5 minutes.
6. When finished, allow releasing pressure naturally then open the lid.
7. Add lime juice and stir well.
8. Serve and enjoy.

White Bean Soup

Ingredients:

- 4 fresh garlic cloves, minced
- 2 celery stalks, diced
- 2 fresh onion , chopped
- 2 tbsp. olive oil
- 1 tsp. sea salt

- 2 cups white beans, rinsed
- 1/2 tsp. cayenne pepper
- 2 tsp. dried oregano
- 1 tsp. fresh rosemary, chopped
- 4 cups filtered alkaline water
- 4 cups unsweetened almond milk

Directions:

1.   Add oil into the instant pot and set the pot on sauté mode.

2.   Add carrots, celery, and fresh fresh onion in oil and sauté until softened, about 6 minutes.

3.   Add fresh garlic and sauté for a minute.

4.   Add beans, seasonings, water, and almond milk and stir to combine.

5.   Cover pot with lid and cook on high pressure for 50 to 55 minutes.

6.   When finished, allow to release pressure naturally then open the lid.

7.   Stir well and serve.

Kale Cauliflower Soup

Ingredients:

- 4 fresh garlic cloves, peeled
- 2 carrots, peeled and chopped
- 2 fresh onion , chopped
- 4 tbsp. olive oil
- 2 cups baby kale
- 1 cup unsweetened coconut milk
- 4 cups of water
- 2 large cauliflower head, chopped
- Pepper
- Salt

Directions:

1.   Add oil into the instant pot and set the pot on sauté mode.
2.   Add carrot, garlic, and fresh fresh onion to the pot and sauté for 5-10 minutes.

3.   Add water and cauliflower and stir well.

4.   Cover pot with lid and cook on high pressure for 20 minutes.

5.   When finished, release pressure using the quick release

6.   than open the lid.

7.   Add kale and coconut milk and stir well.

8.   Blend the soup utilizing a submersion blender until smooth.

9.   Season with pepper and salt.

Healthy Broccoli Asparagus Soup

Ingredients:

- 7 cups filtered alkaline water
- 2 cups cauliflower florets, chopped
- 2 tsp. garlic, chopped
- 2 cup fresh onion , chopped
- 2 tbsp. olive oil
- 2 cups broccoli florets, chopped
- 30 asparagus spears, ends trimmed and chopped
- 2 tsp. dried oregano
- 2 tbsp. fresh thyme leaves
- 1 cup unsweetened almond milk
- Pepper
- Salt

Directions:

1.   Add oil in the instant pot and set the pot on sauté mode.

2.   Add fresh onion to the olive oil and sauté until fresh onion is softened.

3.   Add fresh garlic and sauté for 45 seconds.

4.   Add all vegetables and water and stir well.

5.   Cover pot with lid and cook on manual mode for 4 minutes.

6.   When finished, allow to release pressure naturally then open the lid.

7.   Blend the soup utilizing a submersion blender until smooth.

8.   Stir in almond milk, herbs, pepper, and salt.

9.   Serve and enjoy.

Creamy Asparagus Soup

Ingredients:

- 1 tsp. oregano
- 1 tsp. sage
- 4 cups filtered alkaline water
- 2 cauliflower head, cut into florets
- 2 tbsp. garlic, minced
- 2 leek, sliced
- 4 tbsp. coconut oil
- 2 lbs. fresh asparagus cut off woody stems
- 1/2 tsp. lime zest
- 2 tbsp. lime juice
- 2 4 oz. coconut milk
- 2 tsp. dried thyme
- Pinch of Himalayan salt

Directions:

- Preheat the oven to 450 F/ 250C.
- Line baking tray with parchment paper and set aside.
- Arrange asparagus spears on a baking tray.
- Drizzle with 5 tablespoons of coconut oil and sprinkle with salt, thyme, oregano, and sage.
- Bake in preheated oven for 30-35 minutes.
- Add remaining oil in the instant pot and set the pot on sauté mode.
- Put some fresh garlic and leek to the pot and sauté for 1-5   minutes.
- Add cauliflower florets and water in the pot and stir well.
- Cover pot with lid and select steam mode and set timer for 4 minutes.
- When finished, release pressure using the quick release

Directions.

1. Add roasted asparagus, lime zest, lime juice, and coconut milk and stir well.
2. Blend the soup utilizing a submersion blender until smooth.
3. Serve and enjoy.

Chia And Almond Pudding

Ingredients:

- 2 c. unsweetened almond milk
- 1 c. chia seeds
- 2 tsp. organic vanilla extract
- 2 tbsp. maple syrup
- ⅓ fresh strawberries, hulled and sliced
- 2 tbsp. almonds, sliced

Directions

1. In a large bowl, add the first four ingredients, extract and stir to combine well.
2. Refrigerate for about 3-4 hours, stirring occasionally.
3. Serve with the sliced strawberry and almond slice topping.

Amaranth Porridge

Ingredients:

- 2 c. amaranth
- 2 tbsp. coconut oil
- 2 tbsp. ground cinnamon

- 2 c. almond milk
- 2 c. alkaline water

Directions

1. Mix milk with water in a medium saucepan.
2. Bring the mixture to a boil.
3. Stir in amaranth then reduce the heat to low.
4. Cook on low simmer for 45minutes with occasional stirring.

5. Turn off the heat. Stir in cinnamon and coconut oil.
6. Serve warm.

Zucchini Muffins

Ingredients:

- 1 c. almond milk
- 2 tsp. vanilla extract
- 2 c. almond flour
- 2 tbsp. baking powder
- 2 tsp. cinnamon
- 1/2 tsp. sea salt

- 2 tbsp. ground flaxseed
- 4 tbsp. alkaline water
- 1/2 c. almond butter
- 4 small-medium over-ripe bananas
- 2 small zucchinis, grated

Directions

1. Set your oven to 490 degrees F. Grease a muffin tray with cooking spray.
2. Mix flaxseed with water in a bowl.
3. Mash bananas in a glass bowl and stir in all the remaining ingredients.
4. Mix well and divide the mixture into the muffin tray.
5. Bake for 30 to 35 minutes.

Millet Porridge

Ingredients:

- 1 c. millet, rinsed and drained
- 2 1 c. alkaline water
- 4 drops liquid stevia

- Pinch of sea salt
- 2 tbsp. almonds, finely chopped
- 1 c. unsweetened almond milk

Directions

1. Sauté millet in a non-stick skillet for 4 minutes.
2. Stir in salt and water. Let it boil, then reduce the heat.
3. Cook for 30 minutes, then stirs in remaining ingredients.
4. Cook for another 4 minutes.

5. Serve with chopped nuts on top.

Tofu Vegetable Fry

Ingredients:

- 2 small fresh fresh onion s , finely chopped
- 2 c. cherry tomatoes, finely chopped
- 1/7 tsp. ground turmeric
- 2 tbsp. olive oil
- 2 red bell peppers, seeded and chopped
- 4 c. firm tofu, crumbled and chopped
- 1/7 tsp. cayenne pepper
- 2 tbsp. fresh basil leaves, chopped
- Salt, to taste

Directions

1. Sauté fresh fresh onion s and bell peppers in a greased skillet for 6 minutes.
2. Stir in tomatoes and cook for 2 minutes.
3. Add turmeric, salt, cayenne pepper, and tofu.
4. Cook for 8 minutes.
5. Garnish with basil leaves.
6. Serve warm.

Spiced Quinoa Porridge

Ingredients:

- 1 tsp. ground ginger
- 1 tsp. ground nutmeg
- Pinch of ground cloves
- 2 tbsp. almonds, chopped

- 2 c. uncooked red quinoa, rinsed and drained
- 2 c. water
- 1 tsp. organic vanilla extract
- 1 c. coconut milk
- 1/2 tsp. fresh lemon peel, grated finely
- 2 2 drops liquid stevia
- 2 tsp. ground cinnamon

Directions

1. In a large pan, mix together the quinoa, water, and vanilla extract over medium heat and allow to a boil.
2. Reduce the heat to low and simmer, covered for about 30 minutes or until there is the absorption of all liquid, stirring occasionally.
3. In the pan with the quinoa, add the coconut milk, lemon peel, stevia, and spices and stir to combine.
4. Immediately remove from the heat and use a fork to fluff your quinoa.
5. Divide the quinoa mixture evenly into serving bowls.
6. Serve with a topping of chopped almonds.

Buckwheat Porridge

Ingredients:

- 1 c. buckwheat groats
- 2 tbsp. chia seeds
- 20 almonds
- 2 c. unsweetened almond milk
- 1 tsp. ground cinnamon
- 2 tsp. organic vanilla extract
- 4 drops liquid stevia
- 1/2 c. mixed fresh berries

Directions

1. In a large bowl, soak buckwheat groats in 2 cup of water overnight.
2. In another 2 bowls, soak chia seeds and almonds respectively.
3. Drain the buckwheat and rinse well.

4. In a non-stick pan, add the buckwheat and almond milk over medium heat and cook for about 10 minutes or until creamy.
5. Drain the chia sees and almonds well.
6. Remove the pan from heat and stir in the almonds, chia seeds, cinnamon, vanilla extract, and stevia.
7. Serve hot with a topping of berries.

Overnight Fruity Oatmeal

Ingredients:

- 2 c. unsweetened almond milk
- 1/2 c. fresh blueberries
- 2 tbsp. walnuts, chopped

- 2 c. rolled oats

- 2 large banana, peeled and mashed
- 4 tsp. chia seeds

Directions

1. In a large bowl, add all the ingredients except for sliced blueberries and walnuts and mix well until combined.
2. Cover the bowl and refrigerate overnight.
3. Top with blueberries and walnuts and serve.

Banana Waffles

Ingredients:

- 2 bananas, peeled and mashed
- 2 c. creamy almond butter
- 1/2 c. full-fat coconut milk

- 2 tbsp. flax meal
- 6 tbsp. warm water

Directions

1. In a small bowl, add the flax meal and warm water and beat until well combined.
2. Set aside for about 25 to 30 minutes or until mixture becomes thick.
3. In a medium mixing bowl, add the bananas, almond butter, and coconut milk, mix well.

4. Add the flax meal mixture and mix until well combined.
5. Preheat the waffle iron and lightly grease it.
6. Place the desired amount of the mixture in the preheated waffle iron.
7. Cook for about 4 -4 minutes or until waffles become golden brown.
8. Repeat with the remaining mixture.
9. Serve warm.

Buckwheat Pancakes

Ingredients:

2 tbsp. ground flax seed

1/2 c. maple syrup

2 tsp. vanilla extract

2 c. coconut milk

2 tbsp. baking powder

2 tsp. apple cider vinegar

1/2 tsp. sea salt

2 c. buckwheat flour

2 tbsp. coconut oil

Directions

1. In a medium bowl, mix the coconut milk and vinegar. Set aside.
2. In a separate bowl, mix together the flour, salt, flax seed, and baking powder.

3. Add the coconut milk mixture, vanilla, maple syrup, and beat well to combine.
4. In a large non-stick skillet, melt the coconut oil over medium high heat.
5. Place about ⅓ cup of the mixture and spread in an even circle.
6. Cook for about 1-5 minutes.
7. Flip and cook for an additional
8. 2 minute then remove from pan.
9. Repeat with the rest of the mixture.
10.   Serve warm.

Tomato Omelette

Ingredients:

- 2 medium fresh onion , chopped finely
- 2 medium tomatoes, chopped finely
- 2 jalapeño pepper, chopped finely
- 2 tbsp. fresh cilantro, chopped
- 2 tbsp. olive oil, divided

- 2 c. chickpea flour
- 1/2 tsp. ground turmeric
- 1/2 tsp. red chili powder
- Pinch of ground cumin
- Pinch of salt
- 2 c. water

Directions

1. In a large bowl, mix together the flour, spices, and salt.
2. Slowly add the water and mix until well combined.
3. Add the fresh onion , tomatoes, green chili, and cilantro and gently stir to combine.
4. In a large non-stick frying pan, heat 1 tbsp. of oil over medium heat.
5. Add 1 of tomato mixture and tilt the pan to spread it.
6. Cook for 5-10 minutes.
7. Pour remaining oil over the omelette and carefully flip to the other side.
8. Cook for 5-10 minutes or until golden brown and remove from pan.
9. Repeat with the remaining mixture.

Coconut & Nut Granola

Ingredients:

- ⅔ sunflower seeds
- 1/2 c. coconut oil, melted
- 2 tsp. ground ginger
- 2 tsp. ground cinnamon
- ⅛ tsp. ground cloves
- ⅛ tsp. ground cardamom

- 4 c. unsweetened coconut flakes
- 2 c. walnuts, chopped
- 1 c. flaxseeds
- ⅔ pumpkin seeds
- Pinch of salt

Directions

1. Preheat the oven to 480 degrees F. Lightly grease a large, rimmed baking sheet.
2. In a bowl, add the coconut flakes, walnuts, flaxseeds, pumpkin seeds, sunflower seeds, coconut oil, spices, and salt and toss to coat well.
3. Transfer the mixture onto the prepared baking sheet and spread in an even layer.
4. Bake for about 20 to 25 minutes, stirring after every 1 to 5 minutes.
5. Remove the baking sheet from the oven and let the granola cool completely before serving.
6. Break the granola into desired sized chunks and serve with your favorite non-dairy milk.

Tomato & Greens Salad

Ingredients:

- 2 tbsp. extra-virgin olive oil
- 2 tbsp. fresh lemon juice

- 6 c. fresh baby greens
- 4 c. cherry tomatoes

Directions

1. In a large bowl, add all ingredients and toss to coat well.
2. Serve immediately.

Cucumber & Fresh Fresh Onion Salad

Ingredients:

- 2 tbsp. fresh apple cider vinegar
- Sea salt, to taste
- 1/2 c. fresh cilantro, chopped

- 4 large cucumbers, sliced thinly
- 1 c. fresh onion , sliced
- 2 tbsp. olive oil

Directions

1. In a large bowl, add all ingredients and toss to coat well.
2. Serve immediately.

Apple Salad

Ingredients:

- 4 tbsp. extra-virgin olive oil
- 2 tbsp. apple cider vinegar

- 4 large apples, cored and sliced
- 6 c. fresh baby spinach

Directions

1. In a large bowl, add all the ingredients and toss to coat well.
2. Serve immediately.

Okra Curry

Ingredients:

- 2 tsp. coriander, ground
- 1 tsp. curry powder
- Sea salt and freshly ground black pepper, to taste

- 2 tbsp. olive oil
- 1 tsp. cumin seeds
- 1 tsp. red chili powder
- ¾ lb. trimmed okra pods, cut into 2-inch pieces

Directions

1. In a skillet, add in oil and heat over medium heat and sauté the cumin seeds for 45 seconds.

2. Add the okra and stir fry for 2 -2 1 minutes.
3. Reduce the heat to low and cook, covered for 6-8 minutes, stirring occasionally.
4. Uncover and increase the heat to medium.
5. Stir in curry powder, red chili powder, and coriander and cook for 5 to 10 minutes.
6. Season with salt and remove from heat.
7. Serve hot.

Vegetarian Burgers

Ingredients:

- 2 lb. firm tofu, drained, pressed, and crumbled
- ¾ c. rolled oats
- 1/2 c. flaxseeds
- 2 c. frozen spinach, thawed
- 2   medium fresh onion , chopped finely
- 4 fresh garlic cloves, minced
- 2 tsp. ground cumin
- 2 tsp. red pepper flakes, crushed
- Sea salt and freshly ground black pepper, to taste
- 2 tbsp. olive oil
- 6 c. fresh salad greens

Directions

1. In a large bowl, add all the ingredients except oil and salad greens and mix until well combined.
2. Set aside for about 25 to 30 minutes.
3. Make desired size patties from mixture.
4. In a nonstick frying pan, heat the oil over medium heat and cook the patties for 5 to 10 minutes per side.
5. Serve these patties alongside the salad greens.

Eggplant Curry

Ingredients:

- 2 tsp. curry powder
- 1/2 tsp. cayenne pepper
- Sea salt, to taste
- 2 medium tomato, finely chopped
- 2 large eggplant, cubed
- 2 c. unsweetened coconut milk
- 2 tbsp. fresh cilantro, chopped

- 2 tbsp. coconut oil
- 2   medium fresh onion , chopped finely
- 2 fresh garlic cloves, minced
- 1 tbsp. fresh ginger, minced
- 2   Serrano pepper, seeded and minced

Directions

1. In a large skillet, melt the coconut oil over medium heat and sauté the fresh fresh onion for 8-25 to 30 minutes.
2. Add the garlic, garlic, Serrano pepper, curry powder, cayenne pepper, and salt and sauté for 2 minute.
3. Add the tomato and cook for 4 -4 minutes, crushing with the back of spoon.
4. Add the eggplant and salt and cook for 2 minute, stirring occasionally.
5. Stir in the coconut milk and bring to a gentle boil.
6. Reduce the heat to medium-low and simmer, covered for 25 to 30 minutes or until done completely.
7. Serve with a garnish of cilantro.

Rosemary Roasted Yams

Ingredients:

- 6 fresh rosemary sprigs leave removed and finely chopped stems discarded
- Celtic sea salt, iodine-free, to taste
- Black pepper to taste

- 2 c. cubed yams
- 2 tbsp. coconut oil

Directions

1. Preheat your oven to 490degrees F.
2. Mix yams with rosemary and oil in a bowl.
3. Spread the yams on a baking sheet.
4. Bake for 50 to 55 minutes.

5. Adjust seasoning with salt and pepper.
6. Serve warm.

Quinoa & Lentil Soup

Ingredients:

- 4 c. tomatoes, chopped
- 2 c. red lentils, rinsed and drained
- 1 c. dried quinoa, rinsed and drained
- 2 1 tsp. ground cumin
- 2 tsp. red chili powder
- 6 c. homemade vegetable broth
- 2 c. fresh spinach, chopped

- 2 tbsp. coconut oil
- 4 carrots, peeled and chopped
- 4 celery stalks, chopped
- 2 yellow fresh onion , chopped

- 4 fresh garlic cloves, minced

Directions

1. In a large pan, heat the oil over medium heat and sauté the celery, fresh onion , and carrot for 5 to 10 minutes.
2. Add the fresh garlic and sauté for about 1 to 5 minute.
3. Add the remaining ingredients except spinach and bring to a boil.
4. Reduce the heat to low and simmer, covered for 20 to 25 minutes.
5. Stir in spinach and simmer for 5 to 10 minutes.
6. Serve hot.

Burrito Bowl

Ingredients:

- 1 cup brown rice, cook according to the instructions on the package
- 4 green fresh fresh onion s , thinly sliced
- 2 cloves garlic, minced
- Juice of a lemon
- 2 avocado, peeled, pitted sliced
- 2 cups cooked black beans
- 2 teaspoon ground cumin
- A handful fresh cilantro, chopped
- Salt to taste

Directions:

1. Place a skillet over low heat. Add garlic, cumin, salt, black beans, green fresh fresh onion s and simmer for around 25 to 35 to 40 minutes.
2. Divide the rice into individual serving bowls. Serve the bean mixture over it.

3. Place avocadoes. Sprinkle cilantro and serve.

Alkaline Root Curry

Ingredients:

- 1 cup fresh cilantro, chopped
- 2 teaspoons coriander
- 2 inches fresh ginger, sliced
- 1/2 cup lime juice
- Salt to taste
- Pepper powder to taste
- 2 carrots, peeled, cubed
- 2 beetroots, peeled, cubed
- 2 parsnips, peeled, cubed
- 2 celeriac's, peeled, cubed
- 6 cloves garlic, chopped
- 4 tablespoons grape seed oil or rapeseed oil
- 2 medium fresh fresh onion s , chopped

- 2 red chili peppers, chopped
- 4 tomatoes, chopped
- 2 teaspoon ground turmeric
- 4 inches stick cinnamon
- 2 teaspoons cumin seeds
- 2 teaspoons fennel seeds
- 2 cups coconut milk

Directions:

1. Place the root vegetables on a baking sheet. Sprinkle about 2 tablespoons oil over it. Toss well and bake in a preheated oven at 480 degree F for about 20 minutes or until soft.
2. Meanwhile, place a heavy bottomed skillet over medium heat.
3. Add cumin, coriander and fennel seeds and roast until fragrant.
4. Remove from the pan and powder it (slightly rough).
5. Blend together in a blender, fresh fresh onion s , garlic, ginger and chili.

106

6. Place the skillet back on heat.

7. Add remaining oil. When the oil is heated, add cinnamon and fresh fresh onion paste and sauté until light brown. Add tomatoes and cook for 5 to 10 minutes.

8. Add turmeric and the powder mixture and sauté for a couple of minutes.

9. Add coconut milk and the roasted root vegetables. Heat thoroughly.

10. Serve over cooked brown rice or cauliflower rice.

Vegan Healthy Veggie Lentil Shepherd's Pie

Ingredients:

- 1/2 cup almond milk or soy milk, unsweetened
- Salt to taste
- 2 pound potatoes, rinsed, peeled or scrubbed
- 2 tablespoon vegan butter

For the filling:

- 1 cup frozen corn
- 2 tablespoon arrowroot powder
- 2 cup homemade vegetable broth
- 1/2 teaspoon dried thyme
- 2 cup cooked green lentils
- Salt to taste
- Pepper powder to taste
- 2 carrot, peeled, chopped

- 2 tablespoon olive oil
- 2 stick celery, chopped
- 2 cloves garlic, minced
- 2 small red fresh onion , chopped
- 2 cup mushrooms, sliced
- 4 leaves kale, discard hard stems and ribs, chopped
- 1 cup frozen peas

Directions:

1. Place the potatoes in a large pot filled with water, over medium heat. Cook until the potatoes are soft.
2. Drain and place in a bowl.
3. Mash the potatoes with a potato masher.
4. Add salt, vegan butter and almond milk. Mix well.
5. Place a heavy bottomed skillet over medium heat. Add oil.

6. When the oil is heated, add fresh fresh onion s and fresh garlic and sauté until translucent.

7. Add mushrooms and sauté for a couple of minutes.

8. Add rest of the vegetables and thyme and cook until the vegetables are tender.

9. Sprinkle arrowroot powder over the vegetables and mix well.

10. Add broth, a little at a time and stir each time. Add the cooked lentils and heat thoroughly.

11. Remove from heat and transfer into a baking dish.

12. Spread the mashed potatoes over it. Cover with

13. Bake in a preheated oven at 4 8 0 degree F for about 20 to 25 minutes.

14. Uncover and bake for another 25 to 30 minutes until light brown.

Raw Nut Burger

Ingredients:

- 2 cloves garlic, minced
- 2 teaspoons cayenne pepper or to taste
- Salt to taste
- Pepper powder to taste
- Water as required
- 2 cups walnuts, soaked in water for 5-10 hours
- 2 jalapeño, thinly sliced
- 1 cup sundried tomatoes without oil, soaked in water for an hour
- 2 tablespoons miso paste

Directions:

1. Add all the ingredients into the food processor and pulse until you get a rough paste.

2. Transfer into a bowl. Divide into balls and shape into patties.
3. Either fry on a nonstick pan with a few drops of oil or bake in an oven at 490 degree F until brown on both the sides.
4. Serve with alkaline buns with toppings and sauces of your choice.

Chili Tofu Burger

Ingredients:

- 4 tablespoons chili sauce
- Salt to taste
- Pepper powder to taste
- 2 tablespoons extra virgin olive oil
- Alkaline bread or buns to serve
- 2 pounds firm tofu, chopped into small pieces
- 2 green bell peppers, chopped into small pieces
- 2 large fresh onion , finely chopped

Directions:

1. Place a skillet over medium heat.
2. Add oil. When oil is heated, add fresh fresh onion and bell pepper.
3. Sauté until the fresh fresh onion s are translucent.
4. Add tofu and sauté for another 5-10 minutes.
5. Add chili, sauce, salt and pepper. Sprinkle some water if the mixture is too dry.
6. Slit a bun horizontally and place the mixture in between the 2 pieces and serve or serve between 2 slices of bread.

Sunchoke Pecan Sandwiches

Ingredients:

- 2 cup pecans, coarsely ground
- 1 cup olive oil
- Alkaline bread slices as required
- A few butter lettuce leaves
- 2 small red bell pepper, finely chopped
- 2 cup large basil leaves
- 4 tablespoons lemon juice
- 4 cups sunchokes, coarsely shredded
- 2 ripe avocadoes, peeled, pitted, mashed
- 4-6 ripe tomatoes, sliced into rounds
- Salt to taste
- Cayenne pepper to taste
- Freshly ground pepper to taste

Directions:

1. To make the avocado sauce: Add avocado, lemon juice, salt and cayenne pepper into a blender and blend until smooth. Transfer into a bowl.
2. Add bell pepper, pecans and sunchokes into a bowl.
3. Add half the avocado sauce and mix well.
4. Apply the avocado sauce on one side of all the bread slices.
5. Spread the pecan mixture over a slice of the bread. Place tomato slices, lettuce leaves and basil leaves over it.
6. Cover with another slice.
7. Cut into triangles and serve.

Tofu Steak

Ingredients:

- Salt to taste
- Pepper powder to taste
- A large pinch ground nutmeg
- 1/2 cup lemon juice
- 2 pounds firm tofu
- 1 cup cold pressed extra virgin olive oil
- 4 ounces ground almonds

Directions:

1. Chop the tofu into pieces that resemble steak.
2. Add ground almonds, salt, pepper and nutmeg to a bowl and stir.
3. Place a nonstick pan over medium heat. Add about a tablespoon oil and heat.
4. Pour the lemon juice in a wide bowl.

5. First dip the tofu in lemon juice and dredge in the ground almond mixture and place on the pan.
6. Fry until golden brown on all the sides. Add more oil if required.
7. Remove with a slotted spoon and place on paper towels.
8. Repeat the above 2 steps with the remaining tofu.
9. You can fry in batches
10. Serve with a dip of your choice.

Bean Burrito

Ingredients:

- 2 cups cooked black beans, unsalted
- 2 cup tomatoes, chopped
- 1 cup fresh fresh onion s , chopped
- 2 cup homemade salsa
- 2 tablespoons cilantro
- 6 large lettuce leaves
- 6 sprouted tortillas
- 2 tablespoons ground cumin
- 2 green chili, chopped

Directions:

1. Mix together in a bowl, beans, chili, cumin, fresh fresh onion s , and tomatoes.

2. Place a lettuce leaf over each of the tortillas. Place about 1 cup of the mixture over the lettuce.
3. Spread a little of the salsa over it. Roll, warm it and serve.

Vibrant Veggie Pizza

Ingredients:

- 2 sprouted pita bread
- 2 tomato, chopped
- 2 medium green bell pepper, chopped into 2 inch pieces
- 2 medium red bell pepper, chopped into 2 inch pieces
- 1 cup spinach
- 2 fresh onion , chopped
- 2 teaspoons cayenne pepper
- 2 teaspoons Italian seasoning
- 25 ounces vegan mozzarella cheese, sliced
- 4 tablespoons extra virgin olive oil

Directions:

1. Using a brush, apply olive oil over the pita bread.
2. Add the remaining oil to a skillet. Place the skillet over medium heat.
3. Add fresh fresh onion s , bell peppers, tomatoes, seasoning, salt, pepper and cayenne pepper.
4. Cook until the vegetables are tender.
5. Add spinach and cook until it slightly wilts.
6. Place slices of cheese over the crust of the pita bread.
7. Spread the vegetable mixture over it.
8. Bake in a preheated oven at 480 degree F for about 25 to 30 minutes or until the crust is baked.
9. Slice and serve.

Golden Squash, Pepper, And Tomato Gratin

Ingredients:

- 2 clove garlic, minced
- 1 pound tomatoes, sliced
- 2 tablespoons fresh basil leaves, finely chopped
- 1 cup alkaline bread crumbs
- Salt to taste
- Pepper powder to taste
- 2 golden squash or yellow squash, chopped
- 2 small red bell pepper, chopped
- 2 small fresh onion , chopped
- 4 tablespoons olive oil

Directions:

1. Place a skillet over medium heat. Add 2 - tablespoon olive oil.
2. When oil is hot, add fresh fresh onion and garlic. Sauté until fresh fresh onion s are translucent.
3. Add squash, bell pepper, salt and pepper.
4. Cook until the squash is tender.
5. Transfer into a greased baking dish.
6. Lay the tomato slices over the squash. Sprinkle salt and bread crumbs over the tomato layer.
7. Bake in a preheated oven at 450 degree F for about 20 to 25 minutes or until the breadcrumbs are golden brown.
8. Serve hot or warm.

Tomato Basil Stuffed Spaghetti Squash With

Fresh Garlic Almond Cheezy

Ingredients:

- 2 medium spaghetti squash, halved, deseeded
- 2 leeks, chopped
- 6 Roma tomatoes, chopped
- 2 cloves garlic, crushed
- 4 tablespoons fresh basil, chopped
- 2 tablespoon extra virgin olive oil
- Himalayan pink salt to taste
- A pinch stevia

For fresh garlic almond cheese:

- 1/2 cup almonds
- Himalayan pink salt to taste
- 2 cloves garlic, peeled

Directions:

1. To make the fresh garlic almond cheezy: Blend together in a blender, garlic, almonds and pink salt until smooth. Transfer into a bowl.
2. Place the spaghetti squash halves on a baking sheet with its cut side down. Pour about a cup of water. 450 degree F until tender.
3. Meanwhile, place a skillet over medium heat. Add oil.
4. When the oil is heated, add fresh fresh onion and fresh garlic and sauté until fresh fresh onion s are translucent.
5. Add tomatoes and cook until soft.
6. Add basil, salt and stevia. Remove from heat.
7. Blend with an immersion blender until well combined.
8. Remove the squash from the oven.
9. Use a paring knife; gently pull the squash

10.   Add the cooked sauce in it. Top with fresh garlic almond cheese and serve.

Kale Chickpea Mash

Ingredients:

- 4 tablespoons extra virgin olive oil
- 4 tablespoons liquid aminos
- Salt to taste
- 2 teaspoon dried thyme
- 4 cups cooked chickpeas
- 4 tablespoons garlic, minced
- 2 bunches kale, discard hard ribs and stems, chopped
- 2 shallots, chopped

Directions:

1. Place a skillet over medium heat. Add oil.
2. When oil is hot, add fresh fresh onion and garlic. Sauté until fresh fresh onion s are golden brown.
3. Add kale and sauté until the kale wilts. Add rest of the ingredients and cook for a while.
4. Mash with a fork to the consistency you desire and serve.

Delicious Sweet Potato Dry Stew In Slow Cooker

Ingredients

- 1 tsp. yellow curry powder
- 1/2 tsp. cinnamon, ground
- 2 tsp. Celtic sea salt
- 1/7 tsp. chilli powder
- 1/2 cilantro, finely chopped for garnish
- 2 tbsp. extra virgin olive oil
- 6 orange flesh sweet potatoes
- 4 tsp. garlic, crushed
- 1/2 cup coconut sugar
- 1/2 tsp. black pepper, crushed

Directions:

1. Take the sweet potatoes and clean them thoroughly.
2. Dry them off with a kitchen towel.

3. Peel the sweet potatoes and make 2 inch sized cubes.
4. Take a large mixing bowl and add the diced sweet potatoes to it.
5. Now add all the ingredients one by one except cilantro.
6. Mix together well.
7. Take a crockpot or a slow cooker and add the above mixture to it. Select high setting and let it cook for 2-4 hours, or pick low setting and let it cook for 4-6 hours. Ideally the latter option is recommended.
8. Stir occasionally to coat potatoes with the sauce.
9. When done add the cilantro and salt and pepper to taste. Serve hot.

Cauliflower And Sage Mash

Ingredients

- 7 cups vegetable broth
- 2 tbsp. garlic, crushed
- 2 cups fresh fresh onion s , diced
- 2 cups carrot, diced
- 2 cups celery, chopped
- 1 tsp. black pepper, freshly ground
- 2 tsp. apple cider vinegar
- 1/2 cup maple syrup
- 4 cups almonds, raw and roughly chopped
- 2 cup parsley and cilantro, finely chopped
- Salt to taste
- Freshly Ground Black Pepper, for extra seasoning
- 2 cauliflower head, large and chopped into 2 inch florets

- 2 tortilla chips pack
- 2 1/2 tsp. sage, dried
- 2 tsp. rosemary, dried
- 2 tsp. thyme, dried
- 1 tsp. marjoram, dried

Directions:

1.   Wash   the   cauliflower   florets thoroughly and keep them aside to dry.
2.   Once dried, blend the florets in a food processor till a rough and coarse texture is achieved.
3.   The pulsed mixture should look roughly like rice.
4.   Add the tortilla chips to the food processor and grind.
5.   Stop when roughly chopped.
6.   In a spice grinder add rosemary, sage, marjoram and thyme and grind.
7.   If you don't have a spice grinder, a coffee grinder can be used as well.

8.   Add the ground herbs to the vegetable broth.

9.   Take a large saucepan and heat it over medium heat.

10.   Add olive oil to the above pan and heat it. Add garlic, fresh fresh onion s and a pinch of salt and sauté for around five minutes or till the fresh fresh onion s turn pink.

11.   Add diced celery and carrots to the pan and sauté till they turn soft.

12.   Add the cauliflower mixture to the pan and mix.

13.   Now add chips, salt, pepper and vegetable broth to the pan and mix well. Increase the heat.

14.   Bring the mixture to a boil and then reduce the heat to medium. Let it cook for about half and hour with lid closed. Stir occasionally. The final consistency needs to be that of oatmeal.

15.   Take off heat and add vinegar, maple syrup, almonds, parsley and cilantro and salt to the pan. Mix thoroughly.

16.   Season with pepper and salt and garnish with cilantro and parsley. Serve hot.

Raspberry Delight

Ingredients:

- Zest of a lemon, grated
- 6 tablespoons lemon juice
- 25 to 30 tablespoons water
- 6 drops stevia
- 2 teaspoon agave nectar
- 2 cups frozen raspberries + extra for garnishing
- 2 small avocadoes, peeled, pitted, chopped
- 2 teaspoons fresh ginger, finely grated

Directions:

1. Blend together all the ingredients in a blender smooth.
2. Pour into individual dessert bowls.
3. Chill for a couple of hours.

4. Garnish with raspberries and serve with a spoon.

Rhubarb, Beet & Apple Pudding

Ingredients:

- 2 teaspoon vanilla extract
- 1/2 cup chia seeds
- 2 teaspoons agave nectar
- 6 cups rhubarb, chopped
- Juice of 4 apples
- Juice of 2 beetroots
-

Directions:

1. Add rhubarb and apple juice to an oven proof dish and bake in a preheated oven at 4 8 6 degree F for about 45 minutes or until tender. Stir in between a couple of times.

2. Remove from oven and cool until warm.
3. Add beetroot juice, vanilla and chia seeds. Mix well and set aside for just 25 to 30 minutes,
4. Transfer into a blender and blend until smooth.
5. Add a little water if you find the mixture too thick.
6. Taste and adjust the sweetness if desired.
7. Transfer into individual dessert bowls. Chill and serve.

Chocolate Pudding

Ingredients:

- 1 cup honey
- 2 teaspoons vanilla extract
- 1/2 to 2 cup cocoa powder, unsweetened
- 2 cup almond milk
- 4 ripe avocados, peeled, pitted, chopped

Directions:

1. Blend together all the ingredients in a blender smooth.
2. Pour into individual dessert bowls.
3. Chill and serve.

Orange Pudding

Ingredients:

- 1 cup maple syrup or honey
- 4 cups dates, pitted
- 1 cup fresh orange juice or more if required
- 4 cups mashed avocadoes
- 2 oranges, peeled

Directions:

1. Peel the orange segments and deseed. Add all the ingredients into the blender and blend until smooth.
2. Pour into individual dessert bowls.
3. Chill and serve.

Chocolate Truffle

Ingredients:

- 2 cup sunflower seeds
- 2 dozens whole, soft dates, pitted, chopped, soaked in water for a while
- 4 tablespoons vanilla extract
- 1 cup unsweetened cocoa powder
- 2 cup almonds, roasted

Directions:

1. Add all the ingredients to the food processor. Blend well to form dough.
2. Take about a tablespoon of the dough and form into a ball with your hands.
3. Repeat with rest of the dough.
4. Store in an airtight container.
5. Can store in the refrigerator for a week.

No Bake Cookies

Ingredients:

- 4 cups rolled oats
- 2 teaspoons cocoa powder, unsweetened
- 2 cup water
- 1/2 cup raisins
- 2 tablespoons dried cranberries
- 2 tablespoons walnuts, chopped
- 1 cup natural almond butter or any other nut butter of your choice
- 8 scoops vanilla or chocolate protein powder
- 2 tablespoons ground flaxseeds

Directions:

1. Mix together all the ingredients to form dough like consistency.
2. Shape into cookies and place on a dish which is lined with parchment paper.

3. Freeze for a while and serve.

Raw Vanilla Ice Cream

Ingredients:

- 2 teaspoon lemon juice
- 2 teaspoons vanilla extract
- 6 tablespoons coconut butter
- 4 cups coconut water
- 4 cups young coconut meat
- 2 cup dates, pitted, soaked in water for a while
- 1 cup agave

Directions:

1. Add all the ingredients into a blender and blend until smooth.
2. Place in a freezer safe container and freeze.

3. Transfer into the ice cream maker and freeze according into the instructions of the manufacturer.

Strawberry Coconut Frozen Cream

Ingredients

- 1-5 pound frozen strawberries
- 1-3 tablespoons pure maple syrup
- A pinch salt
- 4 cup coconut cream or full fat coconut milk
- 1 teaspoon vanilla extract

Directions:

1. Place all the ingredients in the food processor jar. Blend until smooth.
2. Pour into a freezer safe container and place in the freezer.

3. Freeze for 4-4 ½ hours or until ice cream is frozen.
4. Remove from the freezer at least 25-30 minutes before serving.
5. Scoop out using a scooper dipped in warm water and serve.

Peach Pie

Ingredients:

For the crust:

- 2 cups almonds
- 2 cups dates, peeled, pitted, soaked in water for a while
-

For the filling:

- 2 tablespoons lemon juice
- 1 cup dates, peeled, pitted, soaked in water for a while
- 1 cup pine nuts
- 1 cup young coconut meat

For the peach layer:
- 1-5 peaches, pitted, sliced

Directions:

1. To make the crust: Add almonds and dates into the food processor and pulse until nearly smooth.
2. Transfer into a pie dish and press.
3. Either use as it is or bake in an oven for a while.
4. Next layer with the peach slices.
5. To make the filling: Add all the ingredients of the filling into the food processor and pulse until smooth.
6. Transfer into the pie dish over the peach slices.
7. Chill and serve.

Berry Banana Ice Cream Cake

Ingredients:
- 6 -6 strawberries, halved

For vanilla ice cream layer:
- 2 cup cashews
- 2 banana, peeled, sliced
- 1 cup dates, pitted, soaked in water for a while
- 2 tablespoons coconut oil, melted
- 1 teaspoon vanilla extract
- 2 cups almond milk

For berry layer:
- 1 cup frozen strawberries
- 1 cup frozen blueberries
- 1 cup coconut water
- 1/2 cup dates, pitted, soaked in water for a while
- 1/2 cup walnuts

Directions:

1. To make vanilla ice cream: Blend together all the ingredients of the vanilla ice cream until smooth.
2. Adjust the consistency you desire by adding vegan milk.
3. Lay the strawberry halves all around a pan. Pour over the strawberries.
4. Place the pan in the freezer to freeze for 4-6 hours.
5. To make the berry layer: Blend together all the ingredients of the berry laycr. Pour over the frozen vanilla ice cream. Freeze for 1-5 hours until set. Remove from the freezer about 25-30 minutes before serving.
6. Slice and serve.

Sweet And Savory Salad

Ingredients:

- 1/2 cup of shelled pistachio, chopped
- Ingredients for dressing:
- 1/2 cup of apple cider vinegar
- 1 cup of olive oil
- 2 clove of garlic, minced
- 2 big head of butter lettuce
- 1 of cucumber, sliced
- 2 pomegranate, seed
- 2 avocado, 2 cubed

Directions:

1. Put the butter lettuce in a salad bowl.

2. Add the remaining ingredients and toss with the salad dressing.

Kale Pesto's Pasta

Ingredients:

- 2 bunch of kale
- 2 cups of fresh basil
- 1/2 cup of extra virgin olive oil
- 1 cup of walnuts
- 2 limes, freshly squeezed
- Sea salt and chili pepper
- 2 zucchini, noodle (spiralizer)

Directions:

1. The night before, soak the walnuts to improve absorption.

2. Put all the recipe ingredients in a blender and blend until the consistency of the cream is reached.

3. Add the zucchini noodles and enjoy.

Beet Salad With Basil Dressing

- 2 tablespoons minced fresh basil
- 2 teaspoon poppy seeds
- A pinch of sea salt
- 1/2 cup blackberries
- 1/2 cup extra-virgin olive oil
- Juice of 2 lemon

FOR THE SALAD:

- 2 celery stalks, chopped
- 4 cooked beets, peeled and chopped
- 2 cup blackberries
- 4 cups spring mix

Directions:

1. To make the dressing, mash the blackberries in a bowl. Whisk in the oil, lemon juice, basil, poppy seeds, and sea salt.

2. To make the salad: Add the celery, beets, blackberries, and spring mix to the bowl with the dressing.

3. Combine and serve.

Basic Salad With Olive Oil Dressing

Ingredients:

- 2 large tomato, hulled and coarsely chopped
- 2 cup diced cucumber
- 2 tablespoons extra-virgin olive oil
- 1/2 teaspoon of sea salt
- 2 cup coarsely chopped iceberg lettuce
- 2 cup coarsely chopped romaine lettuce
- 2 cup fresh baby spinach

Directions:

1. In a bowl, combine the spinach and lettuces. Add the tomato and cucumber.

2. Drizzle with oil and sprinkle with sea salt.

154

3. Mix and serve.

Spinach And Orange Salad With Oil Drizzle

Ingredients:

- 2 tbsp. minced fennel fronds
- Juice of 2 lemon
- 2 tbsp. extra-virgin olive oil
- Pinch sea salt
- 4 cups fresh baby spinach
- 2 blood orange, coarsely chopped
- 1 red fresh onion , thinly sliced
- 1 shallot, finely chopped

Directions:

1. In a bowl, toss together the spinach, orange, red fresh onion , shallot, and fennel fronds.
2. Add the lemon juice, oil, and sea salt.
3. Mix and serve.

Fruit Salad With Coconut-Lime Dressing

Ingredients:

- Juice of 1 lime
- Pinch sea salt
- 1/2 cup full-fat canned coconut milk
- 2 tbsp. raw honey

FOR THE SALAD:

- 1 cup strawberries, thinly sliced
- 1 cup raspberries
- 1 cup blueberries
- 2 bananas, thinly sliced
- 2 mandarin oranges, segmented

Directions:

1. To make the dressing: whisk all the dressing ingredients in a bowl.
2. To make the salad: Add the salad ingredients in a bowl and mix.

3. Drizzle with the dressing and serve.

Cranberry And Brussels Sprouts With Dressing

Ingredients:

- Juice of 2 orange
- 1 tbsp. dried rosemary
- 2 tbsp. scallion, whites only
- 1/2 cup extra-virgin olive oil
- 2 tbsp. apple cider vinegar
- 2 tbsp. pure maple syrup
- Pinch sea salt

FOR THE SALAD:

- 1 cup fresh cranberries
- 4 cups fresh baby spinach
- 2 bunch scallions, greens only, finely chopped
- 2 cup Brussels sprouts, stemmed, halved, and thinly sliced

Directions:

1. To make the dressing: In a bowl, whisk the dressing ingredients.
2. To make the salad: Add the scallions, Brussels sprouts, cranberries, and spinach to the bowl with the dressing.
3. Combine and serve.

Parsnip, Carrot, And Kale Salad With Dressing

Ingredients:

- 2 tbsp. minced fresh mint leaves
- 2 tsp. pure maple syrup
- Pinch sea salt
- 1/2 cup extra-virgin olive oil
- Juice of 2 lime

FOR THE SALAD:

- 1 carrot, grated
- 2 tbsp. sesame seeds
- 2 bunch kale, chopped
- 1 parsnip, grated

Directions:

1. To make the dressing, mix all the dressing ingredients in a bowl.

2. To make the salad, add the kale to the dressing and massage the dressing into the kale for 2 minute.

3. Add the parsnip, carrot, and sesame seeds.

4. Combine and serve.

Tomato Toasts

Ingredients:

- 4 slices of sprouted bread toasts
- 2 tomatoes, sliced
- 2 avocado, mashed
- 2 teaspoon olive oil
- 2 pinch of salt
- ¾ teaspoon ground black pepper

Directions:

1. Blend the olive oil, mashed avocado, salt, and ground black pepper.
2. When the mixture is homogenous – spread it over the sprouted bread.
3. Then place the sliced tomatoes over the toasts.

Turnip Green Soup

Ingredients:

- 4 cups bone broth
- 2 medium cubed white turnip
- 2 large chopped head radish
- 2 bunch chopped kale
- 2   Seville orange, 1 zested and juice reserved
- 1 tsp. sea salt
- 2 bunch cilantro
- 2 tbsps. coconut oil
- 2 large chopped fresh fresh onion
- 4 minced cloves chive
- 2-in piece peeled and minced ginger

Directions:

1. In a skillet, add oil then heat it.

2. Add in the fresh fresh onion s as you stir.

3. Sauté for about 8 minutes then add chive and ginger.

4. Cook for about 2 minute.

5. Add in the turnip, broth, and radish then stir.

6. Bring the soup to boil then reduce the heat to allow it to simmer.

7. Cook for an extra 30 minutes then turn off the heat.

8. Pour in the remaining ingredients.

9. Using a handheld blender, pour the mixture.

10. Garnish with cilantro.

11. Serve warm.

Lentil Kale Soup

Ingredients:

- 2 tsp. dried vegetable broth powder
- 2 tsp. Sazon seasoning
- 2 cup red lentils
- 2 tbsp. Seville orange juice
- 4 cups alkaline water
- 2 bunch kale
- 1 Fresh fresh onion
- 2 Zucchinis
- 2 rib Celery
- 2 stalk Chive
- 2 cup diced tomatoes

Directions:

1. In a greased pan, pour in all the vegetables.
2. Sauté for about 6 minutes then add the tomatoes, broth, and Sazon seasoning.

3. Mix properly then stir in the red lentils together with water.

4. Cook until the lentils become soft and tender.

5. Add the kale then cook for about 2 minutes.

6. Serve warm with the Seville orange juice.

Tangy Lentil Soup

Ingredients:

- 4 finely chopped cloves chive
- 1/2 tsp. ground turmeric
- Sea salt
- Topping
- 1/2 cup coconut yogurt
- 2 cups picked over and rinsed red lentils
- 2 chopped serrano Chile pepper
- 2 large chopped and roughly tomato
- 2 -1 inch peeled and grated piece ginger

Directions:

1. In a pot add the lentils with enough water to cover the lentils.
2. Boil the lentils then reduce the heat.

3. Cook for about 25 to 30 minutes on low heat to simmer.

4. Add the remaining ingredients then stir.

5. Cook until lentils become soft and properly mixed.

6. Garnish a dollop of coconut yogurt.

Vegetable Casserole

Ingredients:

- 4 crushed cloves chive
- 2 cubed yellow Squash,
- 20 halved cherry tomatoes
- 1 tsp. sea salt
- 1/2 tsp. fresh ground pepper
- 1/2 cup alkaline water
- 2 cup fresh seasoned breadcrumbs
- 2 large peeled and sliced eggplants
- Sea salt
- 2 large diced cucumbers
- 2 small diced green peppers
- 2 Small diced red pepper
- 2 Small diced yellow pepper
- 1/2 lb. sliced green beans
- 1 cup olive oil
- 2 large chopped sweet fresh fresh onion
  s

Directions:

1. Adjust the temperature of your oven to 4 6 0ºF.

2. Mix the eggplant with salt then keep it aside.

3. Heat a greased skillet then sautés the eggplant until it is evenly browned.

4. Transfer the eggplant to a separate plate.

5. Sauté the fresh fresh onion s in the same pan until it becomes soft.

6. Add the chive then stir.

7. Cook for about 2 minute then turn off the heat.

8. Layer a greased casserole dish with the eggplants, yellow squash, cucumbers, peppers, and green beans.

9. Add the fresh fresh onion mixture, tomatoes, pepper, and salt.

170

10. Sprinkle the seasoned breadcrumbs as toppings.
11. Bake for about 2 hour and 45 minutes.

Mushroom Leek Soup

Ingredients:

- 1 tsp. ground black pepper
- 2 tbsp. finely minced fresh dill
- 4 cups vegetable broth
- 1/2 cup coconut cream
- 1 cup coconut milk
- 1-5 tbsps. sherry vinegar
- 4 tbsps. divided vegetable oil
- 4 cups finely chopped leeks
- 4 finely minced chive stalks
- 8 cups cleaned and sliced assorted mushrooms
- 6 tbsps. coconut flour
- ½ tsp. sea salt

Directions:

1. Preheat oil in a Dutch oven then sauté the leeks and chive until they become soft.
2. Add in the mushrooms then stir.
3. Sauté for about 25 to 30 minutes.
4. Add pepper, dill, flour, and salt.
5. Mix properly then cook for about 2 minutes.
6. Pour in the broth then cook to boil.
7. Reduce the heat in the oven then add the remaining ingredients.
8. Serve warm with coconut flour bread.

Red Lentil Squash Soup

Ingredients:

- 2 chopped yellow fresh fresh onion
- 2 tsps. dried sage
- 8 cups vegetable broth
- Mineral sea salt and white or fresh cracked pepper
- 2 tbsps. olive oil
- 2 large diced butternut squash
- 2 -1 cups red lentils

Directions:

1. Preheat the oil in a stockpot.
2. Add the fresh fresh onion s then cook for about 6 minutes.
3. Add in the sage and squash.
4. Cook for 6 minutes.
5. Add broth, pepper, lentils, and salt.

6. Cook for about 45 minutes on low heat.
7. Pour the mixture using a handheld blender.
8. Garnish with cilantro.

Cauliflower Potato Curry

Ingredients:

- 2 tbsps. vegetable oil
- 2 cup chopped tomatoes
- 1 tsp. sugar
- 2 florets cauliflower
- 2 chopped potatoes
- 2 small halved lengthways green chili
- A squeeze Seville orange juice
- Handful roughly chopped coriander
- 2 large chopped fresh fresh onion
- A large grated piece of ginger
- 4 finely chopped chive stalks
- 1 tsp. turmeric
- 2 tsp. ground cumin
- 2 tsp. curry powder

Directions:

1. Add the fresh fresh onion to a greased skillet then sauté until soft.
2. Add all the spices in the skillet then stir.
3. Add the cauliflower and potatoes.
4. Sauté for about 10 minutes then add green chilies tomatoes, and sugar.
5. Cover then cook for about 45 minutes.
6. Serve warm with the coriander and Seville orange juice.

Vegetable Bean Curry

Ingredients:

- 2 tbsp. avocado oil
- 2 cans,30 ounces each, rinsed and drained lima beans
- 4 cups cubed and peeled turnips
- 4 cups fresh cauliflower florets
- 4 medium diced zucchinis
- 2 medium seeded and chopped tomatoes
- 2 cups vegetable broth
- 2 cup light coconut milk
- 1 tsp. pepper
- 2 finely chopped fresh fresh onion
- 4 chopped chive stalks
- 4 tsps. coriander powder
- 1 tsp. cinnamon powder
- 2 tsp. ginger powder
- 2 tsp. turmeric powder
- 1 tsp. cayenne pepper

- 2 tbsps. tomato paste
- 1/2 tsp. sea salt

Directions:

1. In a slow cooker, preheat the oil then add all the vegetables.
2. Add in the remaining ingredients then stir.
3. Cook for about 6 hours on low temperature.
4. Serve warm.

Wild Mushroom Soup

Ingredients:

- 1 tsp. dried thyme
- 4 cups alkaline water
- 2 vegetable bouillon cube
- 2 cup coconut cream
- 1 lb. chopped celery root
- 2 tbsp. white wine vinegar
- Fresh cilantro
- 4 oz. walnut butter
- 2 chopped shallot
- 6 oz. chopped portabella mushrooms
- 6 oz. chopped oyster mushrooms
- 6 oz. chopped shiitake mushrooms
- 2 minced chive clove

Directions:

1. In a cooking pan, melt the butter over medium heat.

2. Add the vegetables into the pan then sauté until golden brown.

3. Add the remaining ingredients to the pan then properly mix it.

4. Boil the mixture.

5. Simmer it for 30 minutes on low heat.

6. Add the cream to the soup then pour it using a hand-held blender.

7. Serve warm with the chopped cilantro as toppings.

Bok Choy Soup

Ingredients:

- 2 peeled and sliced zucchinis
- 1 cup cooked hemp seed
- 2 roughly chopped bunch radish
- 2 cup chopped Bok Choy
- 4 cups vegetable broth

Directions:

1. In a pan, mix the ingredients over moderate heat.
2. Let it simmer then cook it for about 25 to 30 minutes until the vegetables become tender.

Conclusion

My opening statement was "Staying healthy is not a matter of chance - it is a deliberate choice." That statement sums up the whole idea of this book and what I have been discussing so far. You can either put yourself in charge of your health by eating healthily, or succumb to the whims and caprices of an uncontrollable appetite which makes you susceptible to every kind of disease and illness.

It is entirely up to you to choose between good digestion and acidifying your system. We do need acids in our body to ensure balance; however, we live in a time and age where a high percentage of what we consume as foods and drinks are highly acidic, causing a shift in the balance that our bodies rightfully deserve. This lopsidedness makes our system overwork itself in a bid to restore its natural balanced state. The result? Too much strain on your body. This can only mean that illnesses are not far away from such a strained body system.

The alkaline diet may be fraught with misconceptions here and there, but no one can deny the efficacy of low-sugar fruits, vegetables, and herbs in general. I have carefully taken a non-sentimental middle path to present to you the very rudiments of how to take advantage of the alkaline diet to improve your overall health and well-being. This is why I have included a comprehensive section about herbs to show you the various ways you can use them as preventive measures against diseases.

Keep this book handy as a go-to guide. That means you'll probably have to read it over and over again, concentrating on sections you need to fully understand or apply. As you do so, do not forget to create a 5 minute daily routine (for at least 30 days) to test your pH level using either your saliva, urine, or both. This is one way that you will know how your body is performing.

www.ingramcontent.com/pod-product-compliance
Lightning Source LLC
Chambersburg PA
CBHW060325030426
42336CB00011B/1209